The Ultimate Vegetarian Salad Cookbook

Easy Vegetarian Salad Recipes For Everyone

Riley Bloom

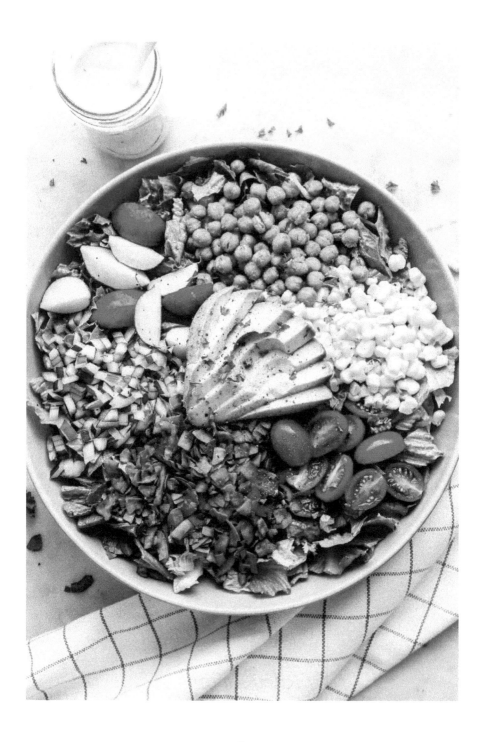

Table of contents

Frisee Lettuce and Two-Cheese Salad

Ingredients:

- 3 ounces pecorino romano cheese, shredded

- 3 ounces cheddar cheese , shredded

- 3 ounces monterey jack cheese, shredded

- 8 ounces vegan cheese

- 6 to 7 cups frisee lettuce, 3 bundles, trimmed

- 1/4 European or seedless cucumber, halved lengthwise, then thinly sliced

- 3 tablespoons chopped or snipped chives

- 16 cherry tomatoes

- 1/2 cup sliced almonds

- 1/4 white onion, sliced

- 2 to 3 tablespoons chopped tarragon leaves

- Salt and pepper, to taste

Directions:

Dressing 1 small shallot, minced 1 tablespoon distilled white vinegar 1/4 lemon, juiced, about 2 teaspoons 1/4 cup extra-virgin olive oil Prep Combine all of the dressing ingredients in a food processor. Toss with the rest of the ingredients and combine well.

Ice Berg Lettuce and Mozarella Salad

Ingredients:

- 3 ounces mozarella cheese, shredded
- 3 ounces cheddar cheese, shredded
- 6 to 7 cups iceberg lettuce, 3 bundles, trimmed
- 1/4 seedless cucumber, halved lengthwise, then thinly sliced
- 3 tablespoons chopped or snipped chives
- 16 small tomatoes
  1/2 cup peanuts
- 1/4 vidalla onion, sliced
- 2 to 3 tablespoons chopped thyme leaves
- Salt and pepper, to taste
- 3 ounces cheddar cheese, shredded
- 3 ounces monterey jack cheese, shredded

Dressing

- 1 small shallot, minced
  1 tablespoon distilled white vinegar
- 1/4 lemon, juiced, about 2 teaspoons

- 1/4 cup extra-virgin olive oil

- ½ tsp. English mustard <u>Prep</u>

Directions:

Combine all of the dressing ingredients in a food processor. Toss with the rest of the ingredients and combine well.

Boston Lettuce and Ricotta Salad

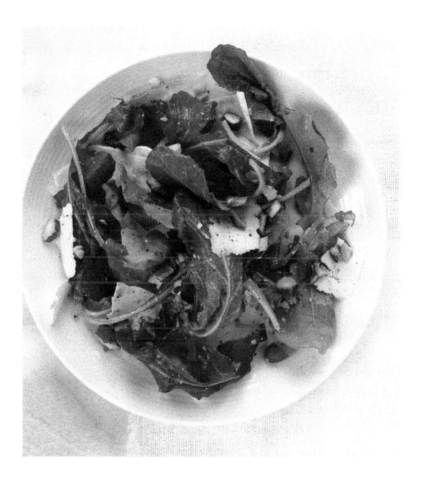

Ingredients:

- 6 to 7 cups Boston lettuce, 3 bundles, trimmed

- 1/4 European or seedless cucumber, halved lengthwise, then thinly sliced

- 3 tablespoons chopped or snipped chives
- 16 cherry tomatoes
  1/2 cup sliced walnuts
- 1/4 red onion, sliced
- 2 to 3 tablespoons chopped tarragon leaves
- Salt and pepper, to taste
- 3 ounces pepperjack cheese, shredded
- 3 ounces ricotta cheese
- 3 ounces cream cheese, crumbled

Dressing

- 1 small shallot, minced
- 1 tablespoon
- distilled white vinegar
- 1/4 lemon, juiced, about 2 teaspoons
- 1/4 cup extra-virgin olive oil
- 1 tbsp. egg-free mayonnaise

Prep

Directions:

Combine all of the dressing ingredients in a food processor. Toss with the rest of the ingredients and combine well.

Romaine Lettuce Tomatoes and Cream Cheese Salad

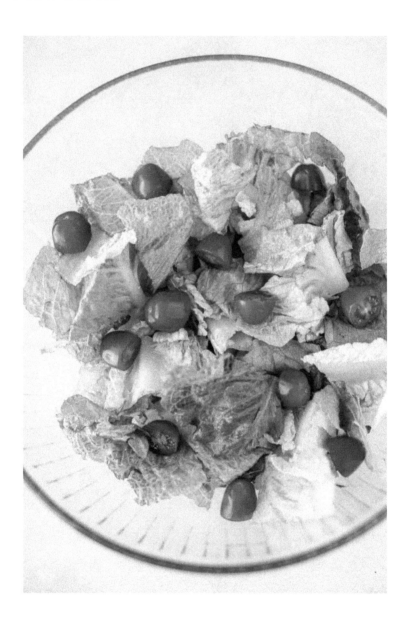

Ingredients:

- 7 cups Romaine lettuce, 3 bundles, trimmed
- 1/4 European or seedless cucumber, halved lengthwise, then thinly sliced
- 3 tablespoons chopped or snipped chives
- 16 cherry tomatoes
- 1/2 cup sliced walnuts
- 1/4 white onion, sliced
- 2 to 3 tablespoons chopped tarragon leaves
- Salt and pepper, to taste
- 3 ounces ricotta cheese
- 3 ounces cream cheese, crumbled
- 3 ounces parmesan cheese, shredded

Dressing

- 1 small shallot, minced
  1 tablespoon
  distilled white vinegar
- 1/4 lemon, juiced, about 2 teaspoons
  1/4 cup extra-virgin olive oil
- Egg-free mayonnaise

<u>Prep</u>

Directions:

Combine all of the dressing ingredients in a food processor. Toss with the rest of the ingredients and combine well.

Stem Lettuce Cucumber and Parmesan Salad

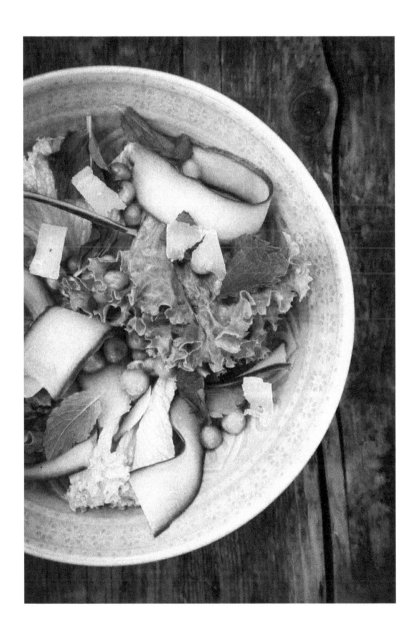

Ingredients:

- 6 to 7 cups stem lettuce, 3 bundles, trimmed
- 1/4 cucumber, halved lengthwise, then thinly sliced
- 3 tablespoons chopped or snipped chives
- 2 mangoes, cubed
- 1/2 cup sliced almonds
- 1/4 white onion, sliced
- 2 to 3 tablespoons chopped tarragon leaves
- Salt and pepper, to taste
- 6 ounces cream cheese, crumbled
- 3 ounces parmesan cheese, shredded

<u>Dressing</u>

- 1 small shallot, minced
- 1 tablespoon distilled white vinegar
- 1/4 lime, juiced, about 2 teaspoons
- 1/4 cup extra-virgin olive oil
- 1 tbsp. honey
- 1 tsp. English mustard

Prep

Directions:

Combine all of the dressing ingredients in a food processor. Toss with the rest of the ingredients and combine well.

Cherry Tomatoes and Pepperjack Cheese Salad

Ingredients:

- 7 cups iceberg lettuce, 3 bundles, trimmed
- 1/4 European or seedless cucumber, halved lengthwise, then thinly sliced
- 3 tablespoons chopped or snipped chives
- 15 cherry tomatoes
- 1/2 cup cashews
- 1/4 white onion, sliced
- 2 to 3 tablespoons chopped tarragon leaves
- Salt and pepper, to taste
- 4 ounces cheddar cheese, shredded
- 3 ounces pepperjack cheese

Dressing

- 1 small shallot, minced
- 1 tablespoon distilled white vinegar
- 1/4 lemon, juiced, about 2 teaspoons

- 1/4 cup extra-virgin olive oil

Prep

Directions:

Combine all of the dressing ingredients in a food processor. Toss with the rest of the ingredients and combine well.

Iceberg Lettuce Apples and Mozarella Salad

Ingredients:

- 3 ounces mozarella cheese, shredded
- 3 ounces cheddar cheese , shredded
- 3 ounces pepperjack cheese, shredded
- 6 to 7 cups iceberg lettuce, 3 bundles, trimmed
- 1/4 European or seedless cucumber, halved lengthwise, then thinly sliced
- 3 tablespoons chopped or snipped chives
- 2 apples, cored and cubed into 2 inch cubes
- 1/2 cup sliced walnuts
- 1/4 white onion, sliced
- 2 to 3 tablespoons chopped tarragon leaves
- Salt and pepper, to taste

Dressing

- 1 small shallot, minced
- 2 tablespoons distilled white vinegar

- 1/4 cup sesame oil

- 1 teaspoon honey

- ½ tsp. egg-free mayonnaise

<u>Prep</u>

Directions:

Combine all of the dressing ingredients in a food processor. Toss with the rest of the ingredients and combine well.

Frisee Cherries and Parmesan Salad

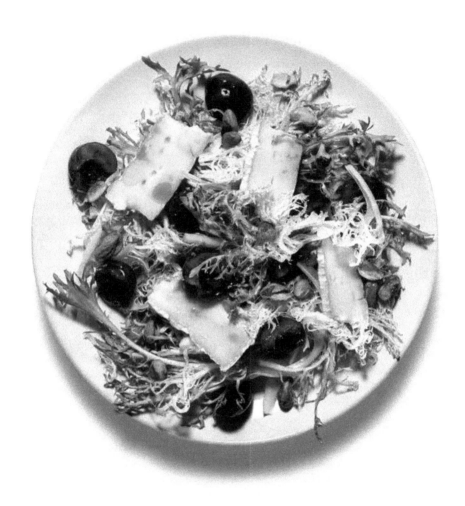

Ingredients:

- 6 to 7 cups frisee lettuce, 3 bundles, trimmed

- 1/4 European or seedless cucumber, halved lengthwise, then thinly sliced

- 3 tablespoons chopped or snipped chives

- 16 cherries, pitted

- 1/2 cup macadamia nuts

- 1/4 red onion, sliced

- 2 to 3 tablespoons chopped tarragon leaves

- Sea salt and pepper, to taste

- 3 ounces pepperjack cheese, shredded

- 3 ounces ricotta cheese

- 3 ounces parmesan cheese, shredded

Dressing

- 1 tbsp. chives, snipped

- 1 tablespoon distilled white vinegar

- 1/4 lemon, juiced, about 2 teaspoons

- 1/4 cup extra-virgin olive oil

- 1 tbsp. honey

Prep

Directions:

Combine all of the dressing ingredients in a food processor. Toss with the rest of the ingredients and combine well.

Romaine Lettuce Cherry Tomatoes and Thai Basil Salad

Ingredients:

- 6 to 7 cups Romaine lettuce, 3 bundles, trimmed
- 1/4 European or seedless cucumber, halved lengthwise, then thinly sliced
- 3 tablespoons chopped or snipped chives
- 16 cherry tomatoes
  1/2 cup walnuts
- 1/4 white onion, sliced
- 2 to 3 tablespoons chopped
- Thai basil
- Salt and pepper, to taste

Dressing

- 1 small scallions, minced
- 1 tablespoon distilled white vinegar
- 1/4 cup sesame oil
- 1 tbsp. sambal oelek

Prep

Directions:

Combine all of the dressing ingredients in a food processor. Toss with the rest of the ingredients and combine well.

Loose-leaf Lettuce Mint Leaves and Cashew Salad

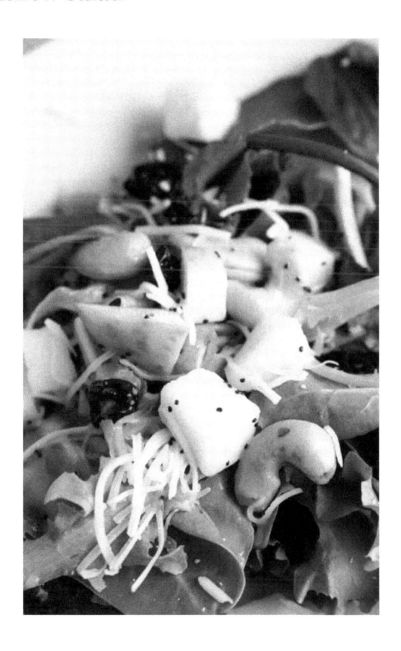

Ingredients:

- 6 to 7 cups loose leaf lettuce, 3 bundles, trimmed
- 1/4 European or seedless cucumber, halved lengthwise, then thinly sliced
- 3 tablespoons chopped or snipped chives
- 16 grapes
- 1/2 cup cashews
- 1/4 red onion, sliced
- 2 to 3 tablespoons chopped mint leaves
- Salt and pepper, to taste
- 3 ounces pepperjack cheese, shredded
- 3 ounces ricotta cheese
- 3 ounces parmesan cheese, shredded

Dressing

- 1 small shallot, minced
- 1 tablespoon distilled white vinegar
- 1/4 lime, juiced, about 2 teaspoons
- 1/4 cup extra-virgin olive oil
- 1 tsp. honey

Prep

Directions:

Combine all of the dressing ingredients in a food processor. Toss with the rest of the ingredients and combine well.

Butter head Lettuce Orange and Monterey Jack Cheese Salad

Ingredients:

- 6 to 7 cups Butter head lettuce, 3 bundles, trimmed

- 1/4 cucumber, halved lengthwise, then thinly sliced

- 3 tablespoons chopped or snipped mint leaves

- 8 slices of mandarin oranges, skins removed and sliced in half

- 1/2 cup sliced almonds

- 1/4 white onion, sliced

- Salt and pepper, to taste

- 3 ounces pecorino romano cheese, shredded

- 3 ounces cream cheese, crumbled

- 3 ounces monterey jack cheese, shredded

Dressing

- 1 small shallot, minced

- 1 tablespoon distilled white vinegar

- 1/4 lime, juiced, about 2 teaspoons

- 1/4 cup sesame oil

- 1 tbsp. honey

Prep

Directions:

Combine all of the dressing ingredients in a food processor. Toss with the rest of the ingredients and combine well.

Romaine Lettuce Tomatoes & Pecorino Romano Salad

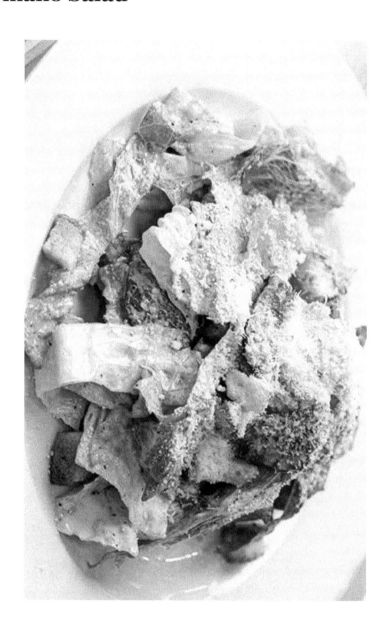

Ingredients:

- 6 to 7 cups Iceberg lettuce, 3 bundles, trimmed
- 1/4 European or seedless cucumber, halved lengthwise, then thinly sliced
- 3 tablespoons chopped or snipped chives
- 16 cherry tomatoes
  1/2 cup hazelnuts
- 10 black grapes, seedless
- 2 to 3 tablespoons chopped tarragon leaves
- Salt and pepper, to taste
- 6 ounces ricotta cheese
- 1 ounces parmesan cheese, shredded
- 1 ounces pecorino romano cheese, shredded

Dressing

- 1 small shallot, minced
- 1 tablespoon distilled white vinegar
- 1/4 lemon, juiced, about 2 teaspoons
- 1/4 cup extra-virgin olive oil
- 1 tbsp. honey

Prep

Directions:

Combine all of the dressing ingredients in a food processor. Toss with the rest of the ingredients and combine well.

Romaine Lettuce Tomatoes Almond and Tarragon Salad

Ingredients:

- 3 ounces pecorino romano cheese, shredded

- 3 ounces cream cheese, crumbled

- 3 ounces mozarella cheese, shredded

- 6 to 7 cups Romaine lettuce, 3 bundles, trimmed

- 1/4 European or seedless cucumber, halved lengthwise, then thinly sliced

- 3 tablespoons chopped or snipped chives

- 16 cherry tomatoes

- 1/2 cup sliced almonds

- 1/4 white onion, sliced

- 2 to 3 tablespoons chopped tarragon leaves

- Salt and pepper, to taste

Dressing

- 1 small shallot, minced

- 1 tablespoon distilled white vinegar

- 1/4 lemon, juiced, about 2 teaspoons

- 1/4 cup extra-virgin olive oil

<u>Prep</u>

Directions:

Combine all of the dressing ingredients in a food processor. Toss with the rest of the ingredients and combine well.

Butter Lettuce and Zucchini with Parmesan Salad

Ingredients:

- 5 ounces cream cheese, crumbled
- 3 ounces mozarella cheese, shredded
- 1 ounces parmesan cheese, shredded
- 6 to 7 cups Butter lettuce, 3 bundles, trimmed
- 1/4 Zucchini, halved lengthwise, then thinly sliced
- 16 cherry tomatoes
  1/2 cup sliced almonds
- 1/4 white onion, sliced
- 2 to 3 tablespoons chopped tarragon leaves
- Salt and pepper, to taste

Dressing

- 1 small shallot, minced
- 1 tablespoon distilled white vinegar
- 1/4 lemon, juiced, about
- 2 teaspoons

- 1/4 cup extra-virgin olive oil

Prep

Directions:

Combine all of the dressing ingredients in a food processor. Toss with the rest of the ingredients and combine well.

Iceberg Lettuce Tomatoes Mozarella and Almond Salad

Ingredients:

- 3 ounces cream cheese, crumbled
- 5 ounces mozarella cheese, shredded
- 6 to 7 cups Iceberg lettuce, 3 bundles, trimmed
- 1/4 European or seedless cucumber, halved lengthwise, then thinly sliced
- 3 tablespoons chopped or snipped chives
- 16 cherry tomatoes
- 1/2 cup sliced almonds
- 1/4 white onion, sliced
- 2 to 3 tablespoons chopped tarragon leaves
- Salt and pepper, to taste

Dressing

- 1 small shallot, minced
- 1 tablespoon distilled white vinegar
- 1/4 lemon, juiced, about 2 teaspoons

- 1/4 cup extra-virgin olive oil

Prep

Directions:

Combine all of the dressing ingredients in a food processor. Toss with the rest of the ingredients and combine well.

Romaine Lettuce Cream Cheese and Pistachio Salad

Ingredients:

- 5 ounces cream cheese, crumbled

- 3 ounces mozarella cheese, shredded

- 6 to 7 cups Romaine lettuce, 3 bundles, trimmed

- 1/4 European or seedless cucumber, halved lengthwise, then thinly sliced

- 3 tablespoons chopped or snipped chives

- 16 cherry tomatoes
  1/2 cup sliced pistachios

- 1/4 Vidalla onion, sliced

- 2 to 3 tablespoons chopped tarragon leaves

- Salt and pepper, to taste

Dressing

- 1 small shallot, minced

- 1 tablespoon distilled white vinegar

- 1/4 lemon, juiced, about 2 teaspoons

- 1/4 cup extra-virgin olive oil

Prep

Directions:

Combine all of the dressing ingredients in a food processor. Toss with the rest of the ingredients and combine well.

Romaine Lettuce with Pepperjack and Feta Salad

Ingredients:

- 6 to 7 cups romaine lettuce, 3 bundles, trimmed
- 1/4 European or seedless cucumber, halved lengthwise, then thinly sliced
- 3 tablespoons chopped or snipped chives
- 16 cherry tomatoes
- 1/2 cup macadamia nuts
- 1/4 red onion, sliced
- Salt and pepper, to taste
- 1 ounces monterey jack cheese, shredded
- 3 ounces ricotta cheese
- 1 ounces cheddar cheese, shredded
- 1 ounces pepperjack cheese, shredded

Dressing

- 1 small shallot, minced
- 1 tablespoon distilled white vinegar

- 1/4 lemon, juiced, about 2 teaspoons

- 1/4 cup extra-virgin olive oil

- 1 tbsp. pesto sauce

Prep

Directions:

Combine all of the dressing ingredients in a food processor. Toss with the rest of the ingredients and combine well.

Frisee Lettuce Tomatoes and Pecorino Romano

Ingredients:

- 6 to 7 cups frisee lettuce, 3 bundles, trimmed
- 1/4 cucumber, halved lengthwise, then thinly sliced
- 3 tablespoons chopped or snipped chives
- 16 cherry tomatoes
  1/2 cup sliced almonds
- 1/4 red onion, sliced
- 2 to 3 tablespoons chopped parsley
- Salt and pepper, to taste
- 3 ounces ricotta cheese
- 2 ounces cheddar cheese, shredded
- 1 ounces pepperjack cheese, shredded
- 1 ounces pecorino romano cheese, shredded

Dressing

- 1 small scallions, minced
- 1 tablespoon distilled white vinegar

- 1/4 lemon, juiced, about 2 teaspoons

- 1/4 cup macadamia nut oil

Prep

Directions:

Combine all of the dressing ingredients in a food processor. Toss with the rest of the ingredients and combine well.

Loose-leaf Lettuce and Pecorino Romano Salad

Ingredients:

- 3 ounces pepperjack cheese, shredded
- 3 ounces pecorino romano cheese, shredded
- 3 ounces cream cheese, crumbled
- 3 ounces mozarella cheese, shredded
- 6 to 7 cups loose leaf head lettuce, 3 bundles, trimmed
- 1/4 cucumber, halved lengthwise, then thinly sliced
- 3 tablespoons snipped chives
- 16 cherry tomatoes
- 1/2 cup peanuts
- 1/4 white onion, sliced
- Salt and pepper, to taste

Dressing

- 1 small shallot, minced
- 2 tablespoon distilled white vinegar
- 1/4 cup sesame seed oil

- 1 tbsp. Thai chili garlic sauce

Prep

Directions:

Combine all of the dressing ingredients in a food processor. Toss with the rest of the ingredients and combine well.

Boston Lettuce Almond and Vegan Cream Cheese Salad

Ingredients:

- 7 cups Boston lettuce, 3 bundles, trimmed
- ½ cucumber, halved lengthwise, then thinly sliced
- 3 tablespoons chopped or snipped chives
- 16 cherry tomatoes
- 1/2 cup sliced almonds
- 1/4 red onion, sliced Salt and pepper, to taste
- 7 ounces vegan cream cheese

Dressing

- 1 small shallot, minced
- 1 tablespoon distilled white vinegar
- 1/4 lemon, juiced, about 2 teaspoons
- 1/4 cup extra-virgin olive oil
- 1 tbsp. chimichurri sauce

Prep

Directions:

Combine all of the dressing ingredients in a food processor. Toss with the rest of the ingredients and combine well.

Mesclun and Tomato with Cilantro Vinaigrette

Ingredients:

- 6 to 7 cups mesclun, 3 bundles, trimmed
- 1/4 cucumber, halved lengthwise, then thinly sliced
- 3 tablespoons chopped or snipped chives
- 16 cherry tomatoes
  1/2 cup sliced almonds
- 1/4 white onion, sliced
- Salt and pepper, to taste
- 1 ounce blue cheese, crumbled
- 3 ounces gouda cheese, shredded
- 3 ounces brie cheese, crumbled

Dressing

- 1 sprig cilantro, minced
- 1 tablespoon distilled white vinegar
- 1/4 lemon, juiced, about 2 teaspoons
- 1/4 cup extra-virgin olive oil

Prep

Directions:

Combine all of the dressing ingredients in a food processor. Toss with the rest of the ingredients and combine well.

Bib Lettuce and Vegan Ricotta Salad

Ingredients:

- 6 to 7 cups bib lettuce, 3 bundles, trimmed
- 1/4 cucumber, halved lengthwise, then thinly sliced
- 16 grapes
- 1/2 cup sliced almonds
- 1/4 white onion, sliced
- Salt and pepper, to taste
- 3 ounces mozarella cheese, shredded
- 3 ounces parmesan cheese, shredded
- 1 ounce blue cheese, crumbled

Dressing

- 1 tablespoon distilled white vinegar
- 1/4 lemon, juiced, about 2 teaspoons
- 1/4 cup extra-virgin olive oil
- 1 tbsp. Chimichurri sauce

<u>Prep</u>

Combine all of the dressing ingredients in a food processor.

Directions:

Toss with the rest of the ingredients and combine well.

Endive Lettuce Tomatillo and Vegan Ricotta Salad

Ingredients:

- 6 to 7 cups endive, 3 bundles, trimmed
- 1/4 cucumber, halved lengthwise, then thinly sliced
- 3 tablespoons chopped or snipped chives
- 16 green tomatillos, sliced in half
- 1/2 cup sliced almonds
- 1/4 white onion, sliced
- Salt and pepper, to taste
- 3 ounces pecorino romano cheese, shredded
- 3 ounces cream cheese, crumbled
- 3 ounces camembert cheese, crumbled

Dressing

- 1 tablespoon distilled white vinegar
- 1/4 lemon, juiced, about 2 teaspoons
- 1/4 cup extra-virgin olive oil
- 1 tsp. Dijon mustard

Prep

Directions:

Combine all of the dressing ingredients in a food processor. Toss with the rest of the ingredients and combine well.

Lettuce Tomatillos and Almond Salad

Ingredients:

- 6 to 7 cups lettuce, 3 bundles, trimmed
- 1/4 cucumber, halved lengthwise, then thinly sliced
- 3 tablespoons chopped or snipped chives
- 16 tomatillos, sliced in half
- 1/2 cup sliced almonds
- 1/4 white onion, sliced
- Salt and pepper, to taste
- 3 ounces cream cheese, crumbled
- 3 ounces camembert cheese, crumbled
- 3 ounces mozarella cheese, shredded

Dressing

- 1 sprig cilantro, minced
- 1 tablespoon distilled white vinegar
- 1/4 lemon, juiced, about 2 teaspoons
- 1/4 cup extra-virgin olive oil
- 1 tsp. English mustard

<u>Prep</u>

Directions:

Combine all of the dressing ingredients in a food processor. Toss with the rest of the ingredients and combine well.

Kale Almond and Vegan Ricotta Salad

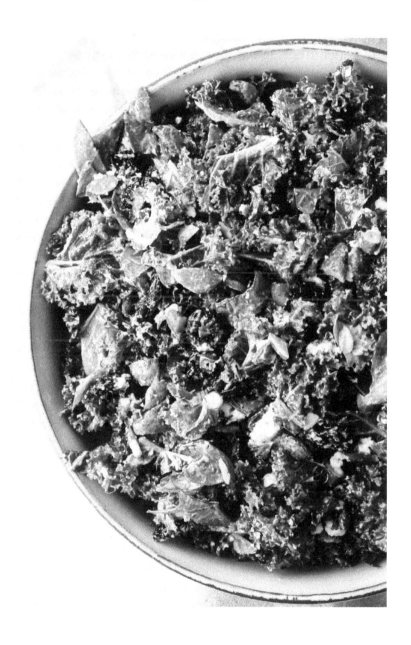

Ingredients:

- 6 to 7 cups kale, 3 bundles, trimmed
- 1/4 cucumber, halved lengthwise, then thinly sliced
- 3 tablespoons chopped or snipped chives
- 16 green tomatillos, sliced in half
  1/2 cup sliced almonds
- 1/4 white onion, sliced
- Salt and pepper, to taste
- 3 ounces cottage cheese, crumbled
- 3 ounces pepperjack cheese, shredded
- 3 ounces pecorino romano cheese, shredded

Dressing

- 1 tablespoon distilled white vinegar
- 1/4 lemon, juiced, about 2 teaspoons
- 1/4 cup extra-virgin olive oil
- 1 tsp. Dijon mustard

<u>Prep</u>

Combine all of the dressing ingredients in a food processor.

Directions:

Toss with the rest of the ingredients and combine well.

Mesclun Tomatillo and Almond Salad

Ingredients:

- 6 to 7 cups mesclun, 3 bundles, trimmed
- 1/4 cucumber, halved lengthwise, then thinly sliced
- 3 tablespoons chopped or snipped chives
- 16 tomatillos, sliced in half
- 1/2 cup sliced almonds
- 1/4 white onion, sliced
- Salt and pepper, to taste
- 3 ounces feta cheese, crumbled
- 3 ounces ricotta cheese
- 3 ounces cheddar cheese, shredded

Dressing

- 1 tablespoon distilled white vinegar
- 1/4 lemon, juiced, about 2 teaspoons
- 1/4 cup extra-virgin olive oil
- 1 tsp. egg-free mayonnaise

Prep

Directions:

Combine all of the dressing ingredients in a food processor. Toss with the rest of the ingredients and combine well.

Bib Lettuce Tomatillo and Almond Salad

Ingredients:

- 6 to 7 cups bib lettuce, 3 bundles, trimmed
- 1/4 cucumber, halved lengthwise, then thinly sliced
- 3 tablespoons chopped or snipped chives
- 16 tomatillos, sliced in half
- 1/2 cup sliced almonds
- 1/4 white onion, sliced
- Salt and pepper, to taste
- 3 ounces monterey jack cheese, shredded
- 3 ounces feta cheese, crumbled

3 ounces ricotta cheese

Dressing

- 1 tablespoon distilled white vinegar
- 1/4 lemon, juiced, about 2 teaspoons
- 1/4 cup extra-virgin olive oil
- 1 tsp. Dijon mustard

Prep

Directions:

Combine all of the dressing ingredients in a food processor. Toss with the rest of the ingredients and combine well.

Butter Lettuce and Feta Cheese Salad

Ingredients:

6 to 7 cups butter lettuce, 3 bundles, trimmed

1/4 cucumber, halved lengthwise, then thinly sliced

3 tablespoons chopped or snipped chives

16 tomatillos, sliced in half

1/2 cup sliced almonds

1/4 white onion, sliced

Salt and pepper, to taste

6 ounces monterey jack cheese, shredded

3 ounces feta cheese, crumbled

Dressing

1 sprig cilantro, minced

1 tablespoon distilled white vinegar

1/4 lemon, juiced, about 2 teaspoons

1/4 cup extra-virgin olive oil

1 tsp. egg free mayonnaise

Prep

Combine all of the dressing ingredients in a food processor.

Directions:

Toss with the rest of the ingredients and combine well.

Mesclun Tomatillo and Cottage Cheese Salad

Ingredients:

- 6 to 7 cups mesclun, 3 bundles, trimmed
- 1/4 cucumber, halved lengthwise, then thinly sliced
- 3 tablespoons chopped or snipped chives
- 16 green tomatillos, sliced in half
- 1/2 cup sliced almonds
- 1/4 white onion, sliced
- Salt and pepper, to taste
- 5 ounces cottage cheese, crumbled
- 3 ounces pepperjack cheese, shredded

Dressing

- 1 sprig cilantro, minced
- 1 tablespoon distilled white vinegar
- 1/4 lemon, juiced, about 2 teaspoons
- 1/4 cup extra-virgin olive oil

<u>Prep</u>

Directions:

Combine all of the dressing ingredients in a food processor. Toss with the rest of the ingredients and combine well.

Endive Tomato and Ricotta Cheese Salad

Ingredients:

- 6 to 7 cups endive, 3 bundles, trimmed

- 1/4 cucumber, halved lengthwise, then thinly sliced

- 3 tablespoons chopped or snipped chives

- 16 cherry tomatoes
  1/2 cup sliced almonds

- 1/4 white onion, sliced

- Salt and pepper, to taste

- 5 ounces ricotta cheese

- 3 ounces cheddar cheese, shredded

Dressing

- 1 sprig cilantro, minced

- 1 tablespoon distilled white vinegar

- 1/4 lemon, juiced, about 2 teaspoons

- 1/4 cup extra-virgin olive oil

- 1 tsp. egg free mayonnaise

Prep

Directions:

Combine all of the dressing ingredients in a food processor. Toss with the rest of the ingredients and combine well.

Kale Cucumber Tomatillo and Camambert Salad

Ingredients:

- 6 to 7 cups kale, 3 bundles, trimmed
- 1/4 cucumber, halved lengthwise, then thinly sliced
- 3 tablespoons chopped or snipped chives
- 16 green tomatillos, sliced in half
- 1/2 cup sliced almonds
- 1/4 white onion, sliced
- Salt and pepper, to taste
- 3 ounces cream cheese, crumbled
- 3 ounces camembert cheese, crumbled

Dressing

- 1 sprig cilantro, minced
- 1 tablespoon distilled white vinegar
- 1/4 lemon, juiced, about 2 teaspoons
- 1/4 cup extra-virgin olive oil
- 1 tsp. English mustard

Prep

Directions:

Combine all of the dressing ingredients in a food processor. Toss with the rest of the ingredients and combine well.

Kale Tomato and Pepperjack Cheese Salad

Ingredients:

- 6 to 7 cups kale, 3 bundles, trimmed
- 1/4 cucumber, halved lengthwise, then thinly sliced
- 3 tablespoons chopped or snipped chives
- 16 cherry tomatoes
- 1/2 cup sliced almonds
- 1/4 white onion, sliced
- Salt and pepper, to taste
- 3 ounces pepperjack cheese, shredded
- 3 ounces pecorino romano cheese, shredded

Dressing

- 1 sprig cilantro, minced
- 1 tablespoon distilled white vinegar
- 1/4 lemon, juiced, about 2 teaspoons
- 1/4 cup extra-virgin olive oil
- 1 tsp. English mustard

Prep

Directions:

Combine all of the dressing ingredients in a food processor. Toss with the rest of the ingredients and combine well.

Napa Cabbage Tomatillo and Tofu Ricotta Cheese Salad

Ingredients:

- 6 to 7 cups napa cabbage, 3 bundles, trimmed
- 1/4 cucumber, halved lengthwise, then thinly sliced
- 3 tablespoons chopped or snipped chives
- 16 green tomatillos, sliced in half
- 1/2 cup sliced almonds
- 1/4 white onion, sliced
- Salt and pepper, to taste
- 1 ounce blue cheese, crumbled
- 6 ounces gouda cheese, shredded

Dressing

- 1 sprig cilantro, minced
- 1 tablespoon distilled white vinegar
- 1/4 lemon, juiced, about 2 teaspoons
- 1/4 cup extra-virgin olive oil
- 1 tsp. egg free mayonnaise

Prep

Directions:

Combine all of the dressing ingredients in a food processor. Toss with the rest of the ingredients and combine well.

Bib Lettuce Tomatillo and Vegan Parmesan Cheese Salad

Ingredients:

- 6 to 7 cups bib lettuce, 3 bundles, trimmed
- 1/4 cucumber, halved lengthwise, then thinly sliced
- 3 tablespoons chopped or snipped chives
- 16 tomatillos, sliced in half
- 1/2 cup sliced almonds
- 1/4 white onion, sliced
- Salt and pepper, to taste
- 7 ounces parmesan cheese, shredded
- 1 ounce blue cheese, crumbled

<u>Dressing</u>

- 1 sprig cilantro, minced
- 1 tablespoon distilled white vinegar
- 1/4 lemon, juiced, about 2 teaspoons
- 1/4 cup extra-virgin olive oil

Prep

Directions:

Combine all of the dressing ingredients in a food processor. Toss with the rest of the ingredients and combine well.

Baby Beet Greens Tomatoes and Tofu Ricotta Cheese Salad

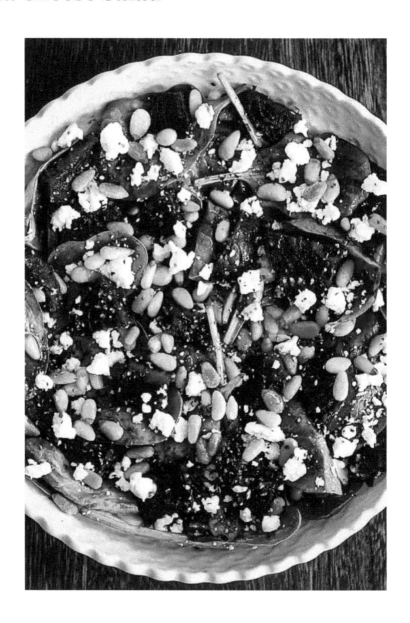

Ingredients:

- 6 to 7 cups baby beet greens, 3 bundles, trimmed
- 1/4 cucumber, halved lengthwise, then thinly sliced
- 3 tablespoons chopped or snipped chives
- 16 cherry tomatoes
- 1/2 cup sliced almonds
- 1/4 white onion, sliced
- Salt and pepper, to taste
- 3 ounces cheddar cheese, shredded
- 5 ounces cottage cheese, crumbled

Dressing

- 1 sprig cilantro, minced
- 1 tablespoon distilled white vinegar
- 1/4 lemon, juiced, about 2 teaspoons
- 1/4 cup extra-virgin olive oil
- 1 tsp. egg free mayonnaise

Prep

Directions:

Combine all of the dressing ingredients in a food processor. Toss with the rest of the ingredients and combine well.

Kale and Cheddar Cheese Salad

Ingredients:

- 6 to 7 cups kale, 3 bundles, trimmed
- 1/4 cucumber, halved lengthwise, then thinly sliced
- 3 tablespoons chopped or snipped chives
- 16 tomatillos, sliced in half
- 1/2 cup sliced almonds
- 1/4 white onion, sliced
- Salt and pepper, to taste
- 5 ounces monterey jack cheese, shredded
- 3 ounces cheddar cheese, shredded

Dressing

- 1 sprig cilantro, minced
- 1 tablespoon distilled white vinegar
- 1/4 lemon, juiced, about 2 teaspoons
- 1/4 cup extra-virgin olive oil
- 1 tsp. English mustard

Prep

Directions:

Combine all of the dressing ingredients in a food processor. Toss with the rest of the ingredients and combine well.

Easy Romaine Lettuce Salad

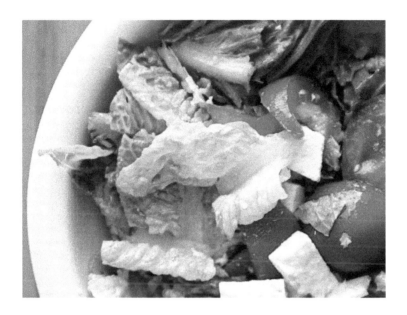

Ingredients:

- 1 head romaine lettuce, rinsed, patted and shredded

Dressing

- 2 tbsp. white wine vinegar

- 4 tablespoons macadamia oil

- Freshly ground black pepper

- 3/4 cup finely ground peanuts

- Sea salt

Prep

Directions:

Combine all of the dressing ingredients in a food processor. Toss with the rest of the ingredients and combine well.

Easy Boston Lettuce and Hazelnut Salad

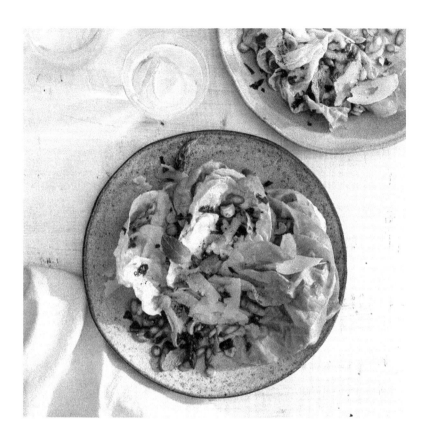

Ingredients:

- Handful of Boston Lettuce, rinsed, patted and shredded

Dressing

- 2 tbsp. apple cider vinegar

- 4 tablespoons olive oil

- Freshly ground black pepper

- 3/4 cup finely coarsely ground hazelnuts

- Sea salt

Directions:

Combine all of the dressing ingredients in a food processor. Toss with the rest of the ingredients and combine well.

Bib Lettuce Salad with Balsamic Glaze

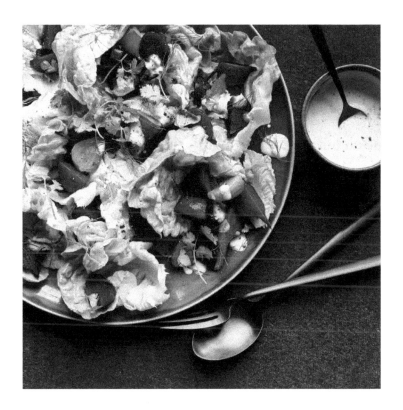

Ingredients:

- 1 head bib lettuce, rinsed, patted and shredded

Dressing

- 2 tbsp. balsamic vinegar

- 4 tablespoons macadamia oil

- Freshly ground black pepper

- 3/4 cup finely ground almonds
- Sea salt

Directions:

Combine all of the dressing ingredients in a food processor. Toss with the rest of the ingredients and combine well.

Mixed Greens Salad

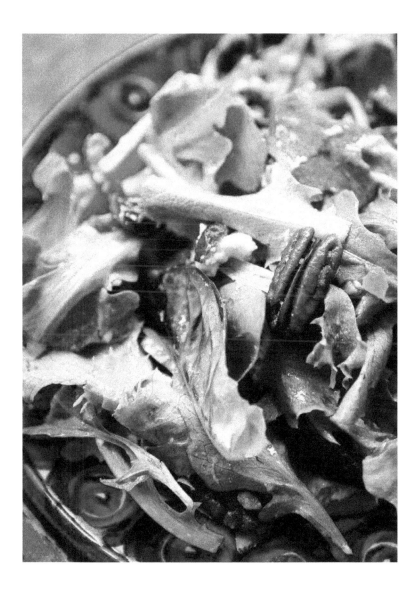

Ingredients:

- Handful of Mesclun, rinsed, patted and shredded

<u>Dressing</u>

- 2 tbsp. distilled white vinegar

- 4 tablespoons extra virgin olive oil

- Freshly ground black pepper

- 3/4 cup finely coarsely ground cashews

- Sea salt

Directions:

Combine all of the dressing ingredients in a food processor. Toss with the rest of the ingredients and combine well.

Boston Lettuce with Cheddar Cheese and Balsamic Glaze

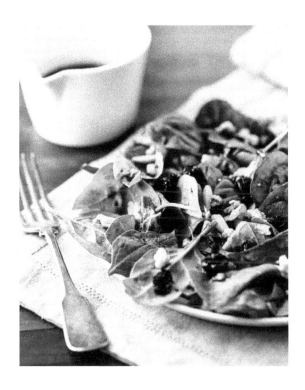

Ingredients:

- 1 head Boston lettuce, rinsed, patted and shredded

Dressing

- 2 tbsp. balsamic vinegar

- 4 tablespoons macadamia oil

- Freshly ground black pepper

- 6 ounces cheddar cheese, shredded

- Sea salt

Directions:

Combine all of the dressing ingredients in a food processor. Toss with the rest of the ingredients and combine well.

Romaine Lettuce with Feta Cheese

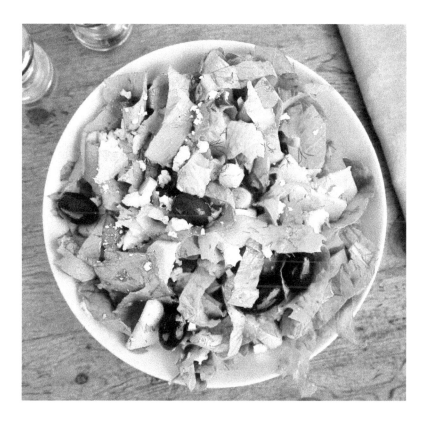

Ingredients:

- 1 head romaine lettuce, rinsed, patted and shredded

Dressing

- 2 tbsp. apple cider vinegar

- 4 tablespoons extra virgin olive oil

- Freshly ground black pepper

- 5 ounces feta cheese, crumbled

- Sea salt

Directions:

Combine all of the dressing ingredients in a food processor. Toss with the rest of the ingredients and combine well.

Endive with Pepperjack Cheese and Balsamic Vinaigrette Salad

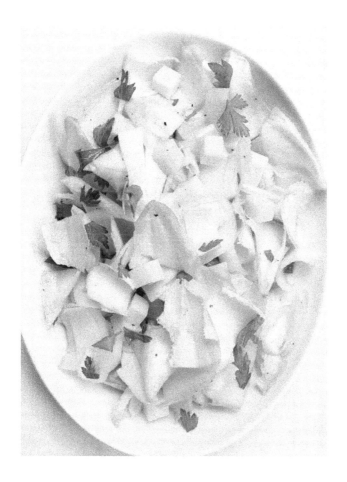

Ingredients:

- 1 Head of Endive, rinsed, patted and shredded

Dressing

- 2 tbsp. balsamic vinegar

- 4 tablespoons extra virgin olive oil

- Freshly ground black pepper

- 4 ounces pepperjack cheese, shredded

- Sea salt

Directions:

Combine all of the dressing ingredients in a food processor. Toss with the rest of the ingredients and combine well.

Bib Lettuce with Walnut Vinaigrette Salad

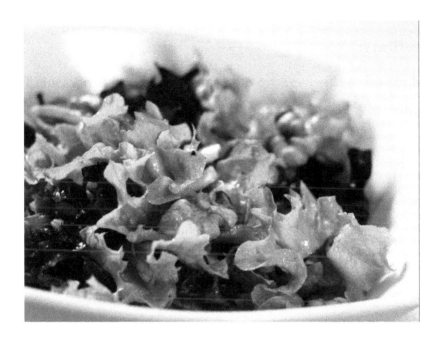

Ingredients:

- 1 head bib lettuce, rinsed, patted and shredded

Dressing

- 2 tbsp. red wine vinegar

- 1 tablespoon extra virgin olive oil

- Freshly ground black pepper

- 3/4 cup finely coarsely ground walnuts

- Sea salt

Directions:

Combine all of the dressing ingredients in a food processor. Toss with the rest of the ingredients and combine well.

Bib Lettuce with Cheddar Cheese Salad

Ingredients:

- 1 head bib lettuce, rinsed, patted and shredded

Dressing

- 2 tbsp. apple cider vinegar

- 4 tablespoons olive oil

- Freshly ground black pepper

- 3 ounces cheddar cheese, shredded

- Sea salt

Directions:

Combine all of the dressing ingredients in a food processor. Toss with the rest of the ingredients and combine well.

Romaine Lettuce with Pepperjack Cheese Salad

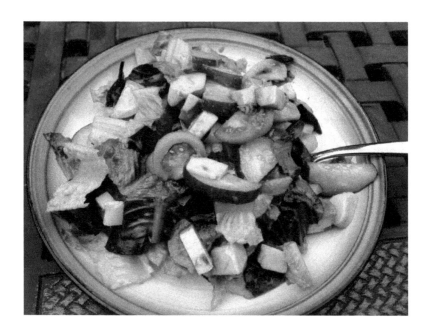

Ingredients:

- 1 head romaine lettuce, rinsed, patted and shredded

Dressing

- 2 tbsp. distilled white vinegar

- 4 tablespoons macadamia oil

- Freshly ground black pepper

- 3 ounces pepperjack cheese, shredded

- Sea salt

Directions:

Combine all of the dressing ingredients in a food processor. Toss with the rest of the ingredients and combine well.

Grilled Romaine Lettuce Salad

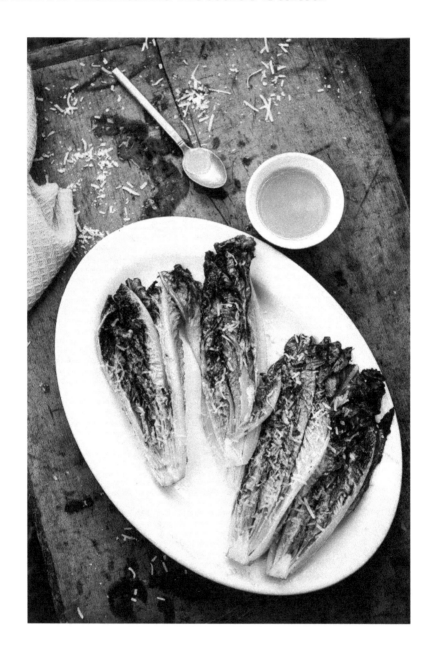

Ingredients:

- 1 head romaine lettuce, rinsed, patted and shredded

Dressing

- 2 tbsp. balsamic vinegar
- 4 tablespoons extra virgin olive oil
- Freshly ground black pepper
- 5 ounces gouda cheese, shredded
- Sea salt

Grill the lettuce and/or greens over medium heat until lightly charred

Directions:

Combine all of the dressing ingredients in a food processor. Toss with the rest of the ingredients and combine well.